Restoring Healthy Heart Rhythms

How I Finally Fixed My Debilitating Cardiac Arrhythmias

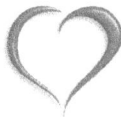

Cameron Powers

Restoring Healthy Heart Rhythms
How I Finally Fixed My Debilitating Cardiac Arrhythmias
First Edition

Original Copyright © 2016 by Cameron Powers
Published by GL Design, Boulder, Colorado, USA

ISBN: 1-933983-26-4
ISBN13: 978-1-933983-26-4
Library of Congress Control Number: 2016906660

Contents

Introduction

Crazy, Out-of-Sync, Palpitating, Erratic and Skipped Heart Beats can lead to a dysfunctional, impaired quality of life. Is there something we can do? Maybe not always, but in my case, yes! Now I have actually begun leading a normal life again! How has this happened? I have finally raised my levels of Intracellular Magnesium. It was not so easy to do. Over the last year I have finally done it and I could feel the gradual improvement all along the way!

Will your Doctors help you? Maybe... But I found that most Doctors don't know how to test you for low "Intracellular Magnesium," which is very different from low "Blood Serum Magnesium."

And unfortunately, most Doctors don't seem to know what it takes to actually fix the extremely common problem of low Intracellular Magnesium. I had to do the research and figure it out myself. And now finally, after 20 years of struggle, I have solid dependable heart rhythms again.

If you are interested in this, don't assume that just by taking some Magnesium pills you can succeed. Keep reading. It can require facilitating Magnesium intake through multiple pathways:

selected foods and water, oral supplements, intravenous infusions, transdermal absorption and reduction or avoidance of certain foods and drinks.

I really think this information might help a lot of people, perhaps including you!

By the way, I highly respect MD's, medical doctors, and am very grateful for their help with my healing. This book is not an attempt to discredit the amazing scientific world of Western medicine. But my own experience has shown that sometimes the doctors are not aware of the simple causes of the most basic health problems. Nor are they always aware of the simplest solutions.

Discovering an effective way to rebuild your levels of intracellular Magnesium can make a critical difference in your health.

Many modern diseases have their basis in Magnesium depletion.

And let me emphasize again right off the bat that the standard blood serum test still used by most doctors will not reveal the truth.

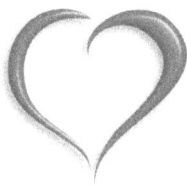

Brief Personal History

My intracellular Magnesium depletion manifested as wild and crazy heart rhythms called "pre-ventricular contractions" and "pre-auricular contractions." "Atrial fibrillation" had been an earlier problem which I will discuss later.

This is not good for a performing musician! This is not good for anybody!

Unfortunately, I know all too well what it feels like to be in the middle of a show and feel my heart rhythm go out! Suddenly my energy sags, brain fog impairs concentration and a feeling of being not well creates a pervasive disorientation and the quality of my musical performance takes a nosedive! Returning again to the Doctors, the Cardiologists tell me that I am just experiencing some harmless "PVC's" or "PAC's". They imply that I am being oversensitive and that I should just live with it.

This is what my heart rhythms looked like for hours every day when my intracellular Magnesium was low...

Sample Arrhythmic EKG

See Below:

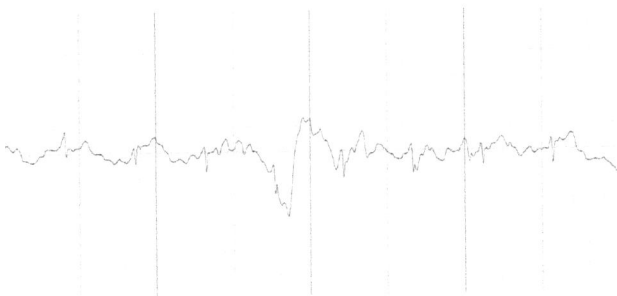

Here is my heart rhythm now steadily back to normal thanks to my intake of Magnesium over a period of months. Intravenous infusions of Magnesium were necessary in my case to make the critical difference.

Sample Normal EKG

See Below:

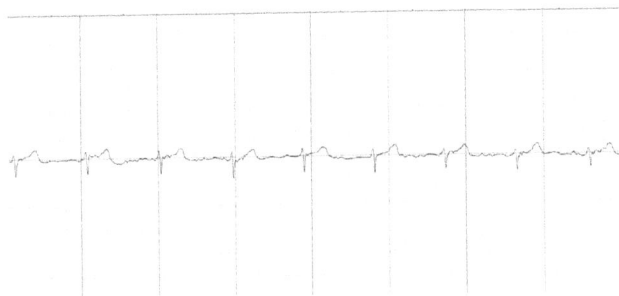

And I also know all too well what it feels like to spend days resting on the couch in such a state of weakness that even just standing up requires a major effort! Trying to just walk to the bathroom causes a further loss of blood to the brain, increased palpitations and a feeling that I am about to faint and collapse! My heart muscle would actually hurt every time the slightest strain was put on it.

Resolving to get to the bottom of these weird heart rhythms, I would head to the Doctors or sometimes to the Emergency Room. Tests were administered and I was given the good news that I am in near perfect cardiac health! This went on for years! I was told that I had no calcifications or hardening of the arteries, no soft plaque, no blockages! Yay! At one point my arrhythmias were so extreme that I was diagnosed with Atrial Fibrillation or "afib" and went through a surgical procedure called Pulmonary Vein Ablation to cure that. But the crazy rhythms called "PVC's" kept coming back. I could actually feel the slight quivering in my heart muscle which triggered the "PVC's" although that quivering never showed up in the EKG's or other tests. I could sometimes slow that quivering feeling with beta blockers so I continued to use them.

So by returning again and again to the emergency rooms and the cardiologists I have eventually had all the heart tests there are to administer! I've passed all the angiograms, CAT scans, treadmill stress tests, EKG's, Holter Monitor tests and Echocardiograms with flying colors! I have virtually no heart disease and none of my arrhythmias are dangerous! Wow!

That's great news! So how come my feet are swelling with edema and my brain is getting so little blood I can hardly think or function? How come I literally feel sick with weakness from the inside out? How come none of those medical experts ever suggested low Intracellular Magnesium? To find out, read on!

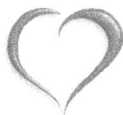

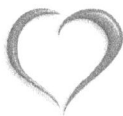

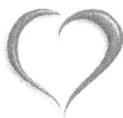

Another Personal History
- Someone Else's Testimony:

"Hi, I am a 50 year old male from South Africa. I never experienced any heart problems until about six months ago. Suddenly I felt extreme heart palpitations – about once every 9th beat – It feels like you're missing a beat but apparently you actually have an extra heartbeat when this happens. I went to the doctors, did tests on everything – no clear evidence of heart problems. No Doctor ever mentioned the possibility of Magnesium deficiency!!?? Are they deliberate in this or have they not been properly educated during their studies? I eventually got onto the internet and decided to try slow-releasing Magnesium capsules. I take 1000Magnesium before I go to sleep. It took about 2weeks but the palpitations stopped completely, totally! And I am not kidding! I had severe palpitations every day during the day and during the night! I will forever stay on this product. I feel more alert as well. It seems funny to me that the medical world tries to steer us clear from Magnesium. Are they crazy not to even mention this if your heart rhythm is failing?? Anyway if you really experience heart palpitations, have it checked as it could be the result of a heart problem like a defective valve. However bear in mind it could possibly just be caused by Magnesium deficiency which is more likely and so easy to solve!!! Hope this helped someone. I'm no expert but this changed my life back to normal functioning. I actually thought I was done for!"

******

Interestingly, my pulse also frequently missed every 9th or 10th beat, just like his! And I also felt like my life was over.

It's great that he fixed his deficiency with oral supplements and without suffering too much from Magnesium's laxative effect, but I needed a lot more Magnesium than we can gain orally to fix my arrhythmias.

Low Intracellular Magnesium May Be Everyone's Problem

Researchers claim that something like 85% of us are low in intracellular Magnesium and that a lot of us are having mysterious health problems as a result.

So I have every reason to believe that the knowledge gained along my healing path could be of use to hundreds of millions of other people!

My Intracellular Magnesium deficiency was manifesting as heart arrhythmias but there are dozens of other common manifestations too!

Multiple Symptoms
of Low Intracellular Magnesium

Early signs of Magnesium deficiency include loss of appetite, headache, nausea, fatigue, and weakness.

More advanced deficiency signs include:

Type II diabetes
Chronic fatigue syndrome
Cardiac arrhythmias
Supraventricular arrhythmias
Ventricular arrhythmias
Atrial tachycardia, fibrillation
Myocardial infarction
Coronary spasms
Chest pain (angina)
Coronary artery disease and atherosclerosis
Torsade de pointes
Hypertension (High Blood Pressure)
ADHD
Epilepsy
Parkinson's disease
Asthma
Bowel diseases
Colorectal Cancer
Kidney disease
Liver disease
Musculoskeletal conditions (fibromyalgia, cramps, chronic back pain, etc.)
Chronic excessive muscle tension
Nerve problems
Seizures
Involuntary eye movements
Vertigo

Numbness and tingling
PMS, infertility, and preeclampsia
Osteoporosis
Migraine
Cluster headaches
Blood clots
Cystitis
Hyperglycemia
Hypoglycemia
Increased intracellular Calcium
Calcium deficiency
Potassium deficiency
Coldness in extremities
Allergies and sensitivities
Body odor
Frequent cavities or poor dental health
Bad short term memory
Poor coordination
Impaired athletic performance
Insulin resistance
Carbohydrate cravings
Anorexia (poor appetite)
Constipation
Kidney stones
Thyroid problems
Raynaud's syndrome
Electrolyte disturbance
Anxiety and panic attacks
Personality changes
Depression
Sleep problems
Difficulty swallowing
Growth retardation or "failure to thrive" in children
Digoxin sensitivity
Altered glucose homeostasis
Hearing Loss

How Magnesium Functions In Our Bodies

Magnesium is necessary for:

Keeping your metabolism running efficiently:
Specifically in terms of insulin sensitivity, glucose regulation, and protection from type 2 diabetes.
Activating muscles and nerves
Creating energy in your body by activating adenosine triphosphate (ATP)
Helping digest proteins, carbohydrates, and fats
Serving as a building block for RNA and DNA synthesis
Acting as a precursor for neurotransmitters like serotonin

Magnesium is the second most abundant ion inside of cells and, along with Calcium, is critical in regulating the electrical activity of the body, including ALL muscle contractions, heart beats and brain activity. Magnesium is also a crucial factor in over 300 enzymatic reactions that require the mineral to be replaced continually.

Magnesium has not attracted the degree of public attention that has been lavished on its complement/antagonist, Calcium. Yet this public relations failure is certainly not due to any biochemical unimportance of Magnesium.

Apparently it is when the Magnesium inside our cells gets low that the health deterioration begins. It seems that Magnesium needs to be plentiful inside our cell walls while Calcium lives in the fluids in between our cells. As we age, our cell walls get leaky and we lose our intracellular Magnesium. It seems Magnesium regulates the quantities of other electrolytes which must be found in our tissues. So, low intracellular Magnesium can mean low Calcium, Sodium or Potassium too.

Or in more technical language:
Magnesium is essential in the glycolytic cycle that converts sugar to ATP (adenosine triphosphate) bioenergy. Magnesium helps stabilize ATP; indeed 80 percent of the Magnesium inside the cell is complexed with ATP. Magnesium is intimately involved in nucleic acid metabolism and the synthesis of DNA and RNA. Magnesium plays key roles in the second messenger systems that mediate hormonal effects on cells. Magnesium is a major controller of cellular ion channels, governing the flow of Sodium, Potassium and Calcium in and out of cells.

While physicians frequently use Calcium channel-blocker drugs to treat various ailments, Magnesium has been called nature's physiological Calcium channel blocker. Magnesium plays critical roles in nerve function and in the contraction and relaxation of muscles, including the smooth muscle cells that constrict or relax arteries. In a very real sense, Magnesium is the mineral of life. Magnesium is the center of the Chlorophyll molecule, without which plant life would not exist, and so neither would the Oxygen of our atmosphere, and so neither would we. It is hard to overestimate the importance of Magnesium.

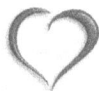

Honestly I must say that discovering my own problem with low intra-cellular Magnesium has given me my youthful energy back. I had reached a point of having to basically give up. I just didn't have the strength to live my life.

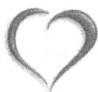

Why are we becoming Magnesium deficient?

A) Our food is being grown in Magnesium-depleted soils. If we were able to drink water straight from streams that flowed over rocks and minerals, or if we ate wild foods rich in Magnesium, none of this would be necessary. But water filtration removes virtually all Magnesium and modern crop-growing methods mobilize as much as 60% less Magnesium compared to older methods.

B) Our ability to absorb enough Magnesium through our stomach and intestines is going down as we age and as other elements like Fluoride and Phosphorus compete for the same biochemical space. The average intake in the elderly drops by 25% or more from the average intake in middle-aged adults.

C) Our tendency to excrete Magnesium through our kidneys increases as we age.

So the first question you will need to answer is, "Am I low on Magnesium?"

Testing For Low Intracellular Magnesium

Most important, of course, is to get the right testing done. Unfortunately, the conversations I have had with half a dozen cardiologists tell me that their training does not provide them with the necessary tools. Yes, they are accustomed to adding Magnesium to their intravenous infusions which they give their cardiac patients, but they think of it as a one-time event. They think that by boosting Magnesium in the blood serum with one treatment that they are solving the problem.

I wondered, of course, how to get tested for low Magnesium. Here it gets tricky. Routine laboratory tests in a hospital or doctor's office often include a Serum Magnesium Level. But the vast majority of Magnesium in our bodies is not IN the bloodstream but in the cells and the fluid surrounding the cells!

Approximately 60 percent of the body's Magnesium is in the skeleton; 39 percent is inside cells (20 percent in skeletal muscle), and less than 1 percent outside the cells (mainly in the bloodstream).Our blood has an amazing ability to keep a balanced Magnesium level at all times, and therefore is the last storage area of Magnesium in the body. So when a hospital test shows a Magnesium deficiency, then it's likely to already be severe and dangerous- with up to 99% of the body's

Magnesium having already been depleted. If you go to your Doctor and ask to be tested it is most likely that your blood will be sent to a lab and the results will come back negative, meaning that your Magnesium is fine. If you accept this diagnosis you may never learn about your true situation.

A serum Magnesium test is actually worse than ineffective, because a test result that is within normal limits lends a false sense of security about the status of the mineral in the body. It also explains why doctors and even most Nutritionists don't recognize Magnesium deficiency; they assume serum Magnesium levels are an accurate measure of all the Magnesium in the body.

Nevertheless, many doctors and researchers believe that Magnesium deficiency is epidemic and in their work with patients, doctors find the lack of a test that can measure clinically meaningful Magnesium levels frustrating.

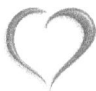

Now here comes the good news!

Although mainstream Doctors and hospital labs may still not be aware of them, there are two tests which can actually determine your intracellular Magnesium levels!

The first test I found about and used is called a 'Sublingual epithelial cell' Magnesium or 'EXA' test. This measures clinically relevant intracellular Magnesium levels painlessly and accurately with only a scrape of a tongue depressor under the tongue. Trial test results show that scrapings of cells directly from the heart wall and from cells under the tongue matched up well for evaluating intracellular Magnesium. My doctor did get Medicare to pay for this $700 test by linking it to my cardiac arrhythmia symptoms.

This sublingual epithelial cell test is not "some test in the experimental stages that we can only someday hope to be able to use in a clinical setting after years of studies and FDA approval."

This innovative test is available to health care providers right now. An additional plus is that it also shows intracellular levels of Calcium, Sodium, Chloride, Potassium and Phosphorus.

A cheaper blood test for Magnesium also exists wherein the red blood cells are centrifuged out of the serum and measured. This is called a Magnesium RBC test. I have been able to confirm the gradual rise of my intracellular Magnesium by using this test, which costs only about $45, as well as by repeating the tongue scraping 'EXA' test which my Doctor was again able to get Medicare to pay for.

Test Results

Here are the results of that first tongue scraping test:

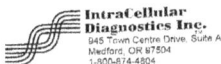

IntraCellular Diagnostics Inc.
945 Town Centre Drive, Suite A
Medford, OR 97504
1-800-874-4804

EXA™ INDIVIDUAL REPORT

INTRACELLULAR LEVELS	RESULTS OUT OF RANGE	RESULTS WITHIN RANGE	REFERENCE RANGES(MEASURED IN mEq/l UNITS)
MAGNESIUM	33.0 L		34.0 - 42.0
CALCIUM	3.0 L		3.2 - 5.0
POTASSIUM		89.6	80.0 - 240.0
SODIUM		3.9	3.8 - 5.8
CHLORIDE	3.1 L		3.4 - 6.0
PHOSPHORUS		15.7	14.2 - 17.0

INTRACELLULAR ELEMENTAL RATIOS	RESULTS OUT OF RANGE	RESULTS WITHIN RANGE	REFERENCE RANGES(MEASURED IN mEq/l UNITS)
PHOSPHORUS/CALCIUM	6.3 H		3.5 - 6.0
MAGNESIUM/CALCIUM		9.4	6.1 - 12.2
MAGNESIUM/PHOSPHORUS		2.1	1.8 - 3.0
POTASSIUM/CALCIUM		20.9	19.1 - 38.0
POTASSIUM/MAGNESIUM	2.3 L		2.4 - 4.8
POTASSIUM/SODIUM	17.9 L		19.4 - 38.9

As you can see, my Magnesium level measured only 33.0 while the normal range is 34.0 – 42.0.

Restoring Healthy Levels of Intracellular Magnesium

Once I discovered that I was indeed low in intracellular Magnesium the game changed: how do I raise these levels? Apparently some folks take the oral Magnesium supplements and restore their health, but I can tell you it's not always so easy to make that work.

It's not so easy but I have found that it can be done by combining the following methods:

1) *Intravenous Magnesium Infusions*
2) *Eating Magnesium-Rich Organic Foods*
3) *Oral Magnesium Supplements*
4) *Magnesium and Calcium*
5) *Enhancing Intestinal Magnesium Absorption*
6) *Reducing Magnesium Excretion*
7) *Magnesium Water*
8) *Colloidal Magnesium*
9) *Transdermal Magnesium*

After feeling my strength deteriorate for twenty years to the point where even trying to stand up from a sitting position triggered such erratic heart rhythms that my life came to a standstill, I have now regained my old sense of solidity and strength and I can function with youthful energy again. I am now 71 years old.

I began with two 1 gram Magnesium infusions a week and could feel the stabilizing effect after two weeks.

After having had more than 20 intravenous Magnesium infusions in the first six months, my intracellular levels were raised enough to make a life-changing difference. I had a much more stable heartbeat but if I let more than 2 weeks intervene between infusions I was in bad shape again.

Now, after having had something like 25 infusions I am experiencing the cardiovascular strength I remember from 20 years ago and can go up to a month without another of infusion.

Test Results

And the second intracellular tongue cell scraping test taken 7 months after the first test revealed that I had moved into the low but acceptable range:

INTRACELLULAR LEVELS	RESULTS OUT OF RANGE	WITHIN RANGE	REFERENCE RANGES (MEASURED IN mEq/l UNITS)
MAGNESIUM		34.9	34.0 - 42.0
CALCIUM		3.3	3.2 - 5.0
POTASSIUM		111.1	80.0 - 240.0
SODIUM		4.2	3.8 - 5.8
CHLORIDE		3.8	3.4 - 6.0
PHOSPHORUS		15.3	14.2 - 17.0

INTRACELLULAR ELEMENTAL LEVELS	RESULTS OUT OF RANGE	WITHIN RANGE	REFERENCE RANGES (MEASURED IN mEq/l UNITS)
PHOSPHORUS / CALCIUM		5.6	3.5 - 6.0
MAGNESIUM / CALCIUM		9.0	6.1 - 12.2
MAGNESIUM / PHOSPHORUS		2.3	1.8 - 3.0
POTASSIUM / CALCIUM		23.6	19.1 - 38.0
POTASSIUM / MAGNESIUM		2.7	2.4 - 4.8
POTASSIUM / SODIUM		20.6	19.4 - 38.9

At 34.9 I am in the lower end of the acceptable normal range of 34.0 – 42.0.
Believe me, I can feel the difference!

And the RBC test on my centrifuged red blood cells which was done 6 months after I began the intravenous infusions shows me at 5.3 (acceptable range 4.2 – 6.8). Different tests measure Magnesium in different units so we must always check our scores against the normal ranges. *(Unless we are professional biochemists or doctors and have in-depth scientific knowledge.)*

Diagnostic Test / Results	Results	Out of Range	Flag	Units	Range
Magnesium, RBC [Final]					
Magnesium, RBC	5.3			mg/dL	4.2-6.8
Tests Performed at Labs / Sites					
LCA_BN	LabCorp Burlington - 1447 York Court Burlington, NC				

It appears that it can take a year of IV infusions to coax the intracellular Magnesium levels back up to where they should be! But fortunately you can be feeling a lot better along the way.

And this is in combination with the other six methods for boosting Magnesium levels which I enumerated!

But whatever it takes is worth it! These Magnesium infusions have given me back my basic life energy!

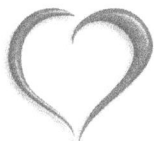

Restoration Methods In Detail

Let me go through the methods I have found for raising intracellular Magnesium in greater detail.

1) Intravenous Magnesium Infusions

My first investigation into raising my intracellular Magnesium led me to what is known as the Myers Cocktail: An intravenous vitamin infusion containing 1 gram of Magnesium Chloride Hexahydrate, multiple B vitamins, and Vitamin C. The infusions are usually given 1-2 times per week, and the most beneficial effects are reportedly felt by the fourth visit.

I found 4 or 5 MDs and Naturopaths near my home in Colorado who offered these. In this case I picked an older MD who ran a straightforward clinic which offered lots of cutting edge integrative medical treatments. I knew what I wanted and found that my initial consultation could be minimal and would only cost $90. The Myers Cocktails followed at $75 per infusion which we began right away twice a week.

I was happy in this case to avoid spending time and money on extensive diagnostics. With this Doctor, who is in his 60's and who has been operating his longevity center for decades, I could establish an easy relationship which left me largely in control. He told me that men my age frequently excrete too much Magnesium through their kidneys and that I might not be able to maintain a normal level of intracellular Magnesium without a long term infusion plan. But he gave me a list of Magnesium-rich foods and educated me about the best oral supplements and encouraged me to imbibe as much Magnesium as possible along with the infusions. He offered me a free 15-minute consultation after every 4th infusion appointment and we covered my questions very efficiently when these came up. I felt very happy with this MD and his friendly staff.

At some point I learned that he offered a larger 2 gram infusion which cost $125 but delivered more Magnesium, Vitamin C and B Vitamins. So I switched to those although receiving that larger quantity did feel slightly systemically overwhelming at times and sometimes I would feel tired the following day. I was told that most people feel that with the larger dose but then feel a stronger and longer positive effect beginning two days later.

Subsequently I found another MD near my chosen healing refuge in the desert in Arizona who offered me the same two options. His introductory consultation was more expensive but could be covered by Medicare.

I've lost track now, but I suppose I've had something close to 30 infusions. And yes, when I feel my heart rhythms start to stray and begin to experience a mild feeling of pain in my heart muscle, I know I am getting low. Two days after an infusion my heart feels good and its rhythms are solid again.

Meanwhile I work on maximizing all my other Magnesium sources and finally seem to be sustaining intracellular levels if I add the intravenous infusions at the rate of one every 5 or 6 weeks.

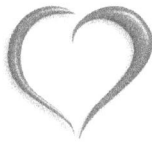

2) Eating Magnesium-Rich Organic Foods

The dietary intake of Magnesium has declined in the United States from 475 - 500 milligrams per day in 1900 to 215 - 283 milligrams per day in 1990, possibly owing to an increase in the consumption of processed foods and the fact that Magnesium is rarely added back to the soil in modern synthetic fertilizers. Pesticides have their negative effect as well. It is difficult to reach the recommended daily allowance of 400 milligrams through diet alone.

Between the mid-1970s and mid-1990s, the USDA tracked the decline of Magnesium in our foods and found a that it decreased by about one third in just that 20 year period alone. If you took the entire food supply grown in the US, assumed no waste and no food fed to animals, and divided it by the population, there would still not be enough to nourish us.

Another researcher in Great Britain also found consistent declines in Magnesium content between 1940 and 1991: Vegetables declined by 24%, Fruit declined by 17%, Meat declined by 15% and Cheeses declined by 26%.

Anyone eating the typical high-meat, high-fat, high-sugar-and-white-flour American diet is likely to have a low dietary Magnesium intake.

Cooking may also diminish the Magnesium content of foods substantially: boiling of vegetables causes a loss of 50 percent of the Magnesium. Spinach and other Oxalate-rich green leafy vegetables are an exception.

Refining white rice into brown rice loses 80 percent of its original Magnesium.

Refined oils remove all Magnesium. The result of oil refining is a zero Magnesium product. Safflower seeds, for example, contain 680 Mg of Magnesium per 1,000 calories. Safflower oil lacks Magnesium entirely.

Refined grains for bread and pasta remove 80-97 percent of Magnesium. At least twenty nutrients are removed in refining flour. And only five are put back when refined flours are "enriched." Magnesium is not one of them.

Refined sugar removes all Magnesium. Molasses, which is removed from the sugar cane in refinement, contains up to 25% of the RDA for Magnesium in one tablespoon. Sugar has none.

It is nearly impossible to get enough Magnesium in your diet from foods alone but you will get the most from Spinach, Chard, Pumpkin seeds, Yogurt or Kefir, Almonds, Black Beans, Avocado, Figs, Dark Chocolate, Banana, Salmon, Coriander, Cashews, Goat Cheese, Artichokes, Navy Beans, Tempeh (fermented soybeans), Pinto Beans, Lima Beans, Kidney Beans, Pumpkin Seeds, Sesame Seeds, Sunflower Seeds, Almonds, Barley, Buckwheat, Brown Rice, Quinoa, and Millet. Many online websites are devoted to providing precise nutritional information.

It seems that among the top ten food contributors to America's total Magnesium intake are items like coffee, beer, and French fries. It's not that these foods are good Magnesium sources. It's just that we eat or drink a lot of them and not much else!

But for those of us seriously trying to eat Magnesium-rich foods, our Daily Values could be met with two servings a day selected from the following: 2 ounces of cashew nuts, 2 cups of boiled or steamed spinach, 2 ounces pumpkin seeds, 2 ounces cashews, 2 ounces of almonds.

We think that getting our minerals like Magnesium in the forms they come through our foods would lead to the best absorption. Well, not necessarily.

In foods, minerals are most often found in inorganic salt forms (like carbonates, chlorides or sulfates). While it is accustomed to dealing with inorganic salt forms, the body's system for transporting minerals can sometimes mis-regulate absorption for minerals that share the same transport channels. An example would be Iron and Calcium, or Zinc and Copper which compete for absorption through the same doorway. Food-forms may not be best at accomplishing higher-than-normal absorption rates. It's much easier for minerals such as Magnesium to hitch a ride with another more easily absorbed compound. So we want to look at oral supplements.

3) Oral Magnesium Supplements

When taking Magnesium supplements, it is important to realize that it may take six weeks to six months to replenish body Magnesium stores through oral supplementation. Thus, if you suffer from many of the listed Magnesium deficiency symptoms and they don't immediately disappear, don't be discouraged and assume they aren't Magnesium-related after all. Just be patient and watch for gradual changes.

Magnesium Glycinate, (also known as Magnesium Bisglycinate), Magnesium Citrate, Magnesium Taurate, Magnesium amino acid chelate, Magnesium Succinate, Magnesium Aspartate, Magnesium Lactate, Magnesium Orotate and Magnesium Picolinate are all absorbable organic forms. Magnesium Chloride is a well-absorbed inorganic form.

Magnesium oxide is the least absorbable and bioavailable form although it may be the most common in health food stores.

The problem with raising your oral intake of supplemental Magnesium is that Magnesium is a laxative. You will have to discover your own limit with how much your intestinal tract can withstand before developing diarrhea. I have found that I cannot tolerate more than about 300-400 Mg/day.

It is best to spread Magnesium supplement intake into at least three daily doses. This will increase absorption and lessen the risk of diarrhea.

4) Magnesium and Calcium Relationship

The relationship between Calcium and Magnesium has been of long standing interest in research. Scientists have long been aware that these two minerals belong to the same family of elements (alkali earth metals), take on the same electrical charge (2+), and have a predictable ratio in different types of soil.

However, only in recent studies have we learned more specific details about Calcium and Magnesium in terms of dietary intake and absorption rate. It turns out that absorption of Magnesium from our intestine depends not only on the amount of Magnesium that is present but also on the amount of Calcium that is present, because the cells lining our intestine have a single spot (called the CaSR receptor) for absorbing these minerals. In practical terms, these circumstances suggest that our diet needs to be balanced in terms of Magnesium and Calcium.

Ideally Magnesium should be taken separately from Calcium, and not with a high-fat meal. If Magnesium is taken with Calcium, it should definitely not be one of the two parts Calcium to one part Magnesium supplements which are commonly sold in health food stores and drugstores. A ratio of 1-to-1 Calcium to Magnesium will be less likely to suppress Magnesium absorption.

Millions of Americans swallow thousands of milligrams of Calcium daily attempting to ward off osteoporosis.

Ironically, research shows that increasing the Magnesium intake improves rather than interferes with Calcium utilization.

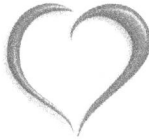

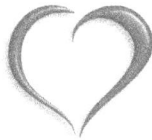

5) Enhancing Intestinal Magnesium Absorption

There are actually some foods and nutrients that aid Magnesium uptake, and conversely, some foods and beverages that inhibit its absorption.

Substances That Promote Magnesium Absorption:

Fructose that occurs naturally in foods like apples, raw honey, dates, plums, and raisins (not to be confused with artificially added fructose).

Complex carbohydrates found in whole grains like oats, barley, buckwheat, and cornmeal.

Protein, especially the alkalizing protein found in whey powder, pumpkin seeds, plain yogurt, quinoa, almonds, and peas.

Healthy oils that contain medium-chain triglycerides, such as coconut oil.
Fruits and vegetables rich in soluble fiber help with large intestine absorption of Magnesium.

Vitamin B6 has been shown to increase intracellular uptake of Magnesium, so it may be useful in getting Magnesium where it belongs: inside the cell.

Cooking releases Magnesium for easier absorption

in certain green leafy foods: The debate about raw vs. cooked foods will probably never be completely settled. But the fact is that some nutrients, Magnesium included, are released from the food matrix through the process of cooking (particularly quick, gentle cooking such as sautéing or steaming). Another benefit of cooking is that it lessens the amount of oxalic acid in foods like spinach. Oxalic acid can hinder Magnesium absorption, and research shows that cooked spinach has a higher Magnesium absorption rate than raw.

Puree Foods To Increase Magnesium Bioavailability: Pureeing foods in your blender is another way to free up Magnesium. Fibrous plant foods can "lock up" Magnesium within their fibers, and pureeing breaks the matrix into such small pieces that the body is better able to extract the nutrients. Basically, pureeing is like chewing in that it mechanically breaks down food.

Substances That Hinder Magnesium Absorption:

Magnesium easily combines with phosphoric acid to make Magnesium Phosphate, which is totally insoluble and precipitates out of the intestinal juices, becoming part of the feces. Americans drink tons of phosphoric acid-containing soft drinks. These Phosphoric acid-containing sodas impair Magnesium absorption by forming phosphates, which bind to Calcium and Magnesium to form an insoluble complex of Magnesium, Calcium, and Phosphate.

Fluoride, like Phosphate, binds with Magnesium in our bodies and tie it up in useless compounds.

Cow's milk, which contains high amounts of Phosphorous, inhibits Magnesium uptake for the same reason as colas.

Oxalates in foods such as raw spinach, rhubarb and chocolate form insoluble Magnesium compounds that cannot be easily absorbed.

Proton pump inhibitors reduce our digestive efficiency and should be avoided. Stomach acid is the second digestive substance that your food comes in contact with (the first is saliva). This acid is required for the proper uptake of many nutrients, Magnesium included. This is why reflux drugs like Protonix, Prilosec, Nexium and other proton pump inhibitors are a problem: no matter how much Magnesium you ingest, your body can't deliver it where it belongs.

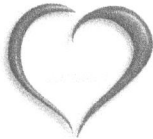

6) Reducing Magnesium Excretion

The main way the body conserves its Magnesium supply is through the kidneys. Healthy kidneys typically reabsorb as much as 95 percent of the Magnesium before it is excreted in the urine. Unfortunately, there are many common factors that promote the kidneys excretion of Magnesium. These include diuretics and digitalis; alcohol; high sugar intake; coffee; high blood levels of the stress hormones adrenalin, noradrenalin and cortisol; aminoglycosides, cisplatin and cyclosporine; and noise stress.

Although the American medical/nutritional establishment promotes Calcium and favors it for mega dosages, high Calcium intake both retards Magnesium absorption and promotes Magnesium excretion in the urine.

Boron is essential for healthy bone and joint function and is responsible for regulating the absorption and metabolism of Calcium, Magnesium and Phosphorus. Boron deficiency causes greatly increased amounts of Calcium and Magnesium to be lost with the urine.

A high-fat diet (the typical American diet is 40 to 45 percent fat calories) may decrease Magnesium retention by 50 percent, even in those consuming adequate Magnesium.

Coffee and tea have diuretic effects which increase Magnesium secretion via the urine.

Excessive alcohol use also inflames the intestines and causes a diuretic effect.

Laxatives also promote intestinal Magnesium loss.

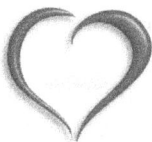

7) Drinking Magnesium Water

Magnesium dissolved in water (ionized) is considerably more bioavailable than is Magnesium in solid tablets or capsules. About 50% of the Magnesium contained in Magnesium Bicarbonate water is absorbed.

Our drinking water can be surprisingly rich in Magnesium, but the Magnesium content of water varies dramatically. Generally speaking, water that is allowed to percolate through Magnesium-rich soil and rock can pick up a large amount of Magnesium. There are bottled mineral waters which have long been prized for their health promoting qualities that provide over 100 milligrams of Magnesium per liter. That level means 25% of the Daily Value (DV) in one liter bottle of water but unfortunately some of these bottled mineral waters are also fairly high in Sodium and Calcium. There are also municipal water supplies in the U.S. that provide nearly 50 Mg of Magnesium per liter but some municipal water supplies contain no Magnesium whatsoever.

Here is a recipe for making drinkable Magnesium Bicarbonate from Magnesium Hydroxide (Milk of Magnesia). I have begun making and drinking this formula and it seems to be helping considerably.

Here are the necessary ingredients:

1) A one-liter bottle of fully carbonated water. Carbonated waters such as Canada Dry Seltzer, which consist of only water and carbon dioxide (CO_2), are suitable. Club sodas such as Schweppes Club Soda are also suitable; they are carbonated water with a small amount of added Sodium.
2) Milk of Magnesia
3) Filtered or Purified Water

To prepare the water follow these four steps:
A) Chill a One Liter Bottle of Seltzer Water to refrigerator temperature

B) Shake well the bottle of Milk of Magnesia, then measure out as accurately as possible 3 tablespoons (45 ml) and have it ready. The plastic measuring cup that comes with the Milk of Magnesia is accurate and ideal for the purpose.

C) Remove the bottle of carbonated water from the refrigerator without agitating it. Open it slowly and carefully to minimize the loss of CO_2. As soon as the initial fizzing settles down, slowly add the pre-measured Milk of Magnesia. Promptly replace the cap on the water bottle and shake it vigorously for 30 seconds or so, making the liquid cloudy. Let it sit back in the refrigerator.

D) After ½ hour or so the liquid will have cleared, and any un-dissolved Magnesium Hydroxide will have settled to the bottom of the bottle. Again shake the bottle vigorously for 30 seconds or so, making the liquid cloudy again. Let it sit again. When the liquid again clears all of the Magnesium Hydroxide in the Milk of Magnesia should have reacted with all of the CO_2 to become dissolved (ionized) Magnesium and Bicarbonate. However, if a small amount of un-dissolved Magnesium Hydroxide still remains in the bottom of the bottle as sediment it may be ignored. This 1 liter of concentrated Magnesium Bicarbonate water will have approximately 1500 Mg of Magnesium and approximately 7500 Mg of Bicarbonate. It should be kept in the refrigerator. You may note that the sides of the bottle "cave in" when the liquid clears. This is a sign that the reaction is complete. This is a concentrated solution which will yield 12 liters of Magnesium water.

E) Measure and transfer 1/3 liter of the concentrate (333 ml) into a 4-liter container. Finish filling the container with 3 2/3 liters of plain or purified water, as desired. This will produce 4 liters of Magnesium Bicarbonate drinking water with approximately 125 Mg of Magnesium and approximately 625 Mg of Bicarbonate per liter and a pH of approximately 8+.

F) Drink It
The alkaline Magnesium/Bicarbonate water should be consumed throughout the day. It can be consumed with a meal, but not in such quantities that it results in dilution of stomach acid. Anyone not in the habit of drinking water should begin by consuming small daily amounts, and should take at least a month to reach a consumption of 1 to 2 liters per day.

8) Colloidal Magnesium

Colloidal forms of Magnesium are available. Although most analysts feel that Colloidal Magnesium doesn't tend to be very well absorbed because it is elemental rather than ionic and therefore inert and non-reactive, others claim that our bodies love it and drink it in.

I ordered some and have been drinking small amounts daily. I have no idea if it is helping me raise my levels of intracellular Magnesium or not, but am optimistically giving it a try.

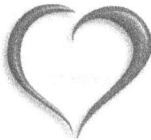

9) Transdermal Magnesium

Many claim that by spraying Magnesium "oil" on the skin and soaking the feet in concentrated Magnesium Chloride baths or by bathing the whole body in "Epsom Salts" (Magnesium sulfate) they can help maintain higher levels of intracellular Magnesium.
It certainly makes sense that we can absorb Magnesium directly through our skin. It makes less sense when we learn that the surface area of the inside of our gut is 7 times larger than the surface area of all the skin on our body.

These transdermal Magnesium supplements are very inexpensive and I have been trying them out. For a while I was very diligent about spraying the Magnesium Chloride (Magnesium Oil) on my skin and soaking my feet in Magnesium Chloride flake foot baths. I concluded that it was not providing as large a contribution as I had initially hoped. But I still persist in spraying the Magnesium Oil on my skin although I have had to learn which parts of my body are immune to the slight stinging effect and spray it only on those.

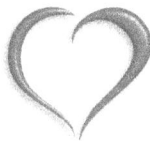

10) Summary of What Is Working For Me

After a year of working on bringing up my Intracellular
Magnesium I am still in the habit of seeking a 2
gram Magnesium Chloride Hexahydrate intravenous
infusion about once a month. But I have been 5 weeks
without one now as I write this so I may have finally
succeeded in maintaining my levels without needing
the infusions. I take 300-400 Mg of Magnesium
Glycinate and drink a liter of Magnesium Bicarbonate
water every day. I eat more organic Magnesium-rich
foods and have reduced coffee and sugar intakes. I
also spray Magnesium Chloride on my skin and take
sips from my bottle of colloidal Magnesium. I also take
Boron, Potassium Gluconate, MultiVitamin, Vitamin
C, Vitamin B6, Vitamin B12, Betain HCL, 5-MTHF Folic
Acid, Tri-Iodine supplements every day. My heart
rhythms are finally solid again. I have no pains in my
heart muscle and can climb fairly strenuous mountain
trails for up to 3 hours a day. I am still rebuilding my
endurance but it is coming back.

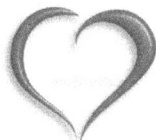

Detailed Personal History

Personal History of Struggle with Heart Arrhythmias and Atrial Fibrillation (Afib):

Twenty years ago in the mid-1990's I began experiences paroxysmal atrial fibrillation. They say that tall men with a history of sustained cardiac exercise are more inclined to develop this problem. So it seemed that all that mountain climbing and cross-country skiing which I had so enjoyed was coming back in a negative way to haunt me. I had no other explanations offered to me.

I frequently ended up in the emergency room where, after trying to use various drugs, the doctors would use the electric paddles to shock my heart back into normal sinus rhythm. It kept working, but the word was that "afib begets afib" meaning the more often the afib happens the more often it's going to happen. Not good news. For years I was on blood thinners and beta-blockers. My ability to plan sustained events in musical performance deteriorated as it proved to be very difficult to continue to function while in afib.

I know that there are a lot of different kinds of heart arrhythmias and you may be afflicted by a different kind or by a different medical condition. But knowing what I know now, I can't help but wonder if they are not all possibly related to low intracellular Magnesium.

I found a pair of doctors in France in 2005 who developed a fairly non-invasive surgical technique called "pulmonary vein ablation" which could cure atrial fibrillation with a success rate of 80%. It was also affordable thanks to the French medical system so I made the appointment and six months later had the procedure. That operation cured the afib and I was able to go off of the blood thinners but unfortunately that didn't cure all of my arrhythmias. In fact for much of the last ten years I have been so out of rhythm with so-called "harmless" PVC's and PAC's (pre-ventricular contractions and pre-auricular contractions) that remaining active and creative has been a real struggle and I finally reached the point of having to cancel all future musical performances. And that quivering feeling in my heart kept stimulating more arrhythmias so I was never able to go off the beta blockers until I was finally able to raise my intracellular Magnesium levels.

As I mentioned at the beginning of this book, I had eventually had all the heart tests there are to administer and was always pronounced healthy. They said they could see my crazy rhythms in the EKG's but that they were not considered dangerous since they were no longer classified as afib. They acknowledged that they might make me weak but they said that they could offer no solutions.

One of my chief cardiologists suggested: it could be that my atrial fibrillation had been actually triggered and maybe even caused by my "harmless" PVC's and PAC's. Now it seems to me that quite possibly my low intracellular Magnesium levels were responsible for those PVC's and PAC's which led to the afib.

How come none of those medical experts ever suggested that low intracellular Magnesium might be a major contributing factor to creating these arrhythmias? And that there might be a solution!

If only I had known!

Additional information on this subject is plentiful on the internet. I leave the search in your hands as I don't want to accidentally appear to be endorsing any particular products or services.

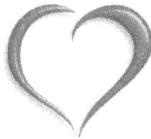

Other Books by Cameron Powers

Naked Wild and Free in the Grand Canyon
Rowing and Roaming

Spiritual Traveler:
Journeys Beyond Fear

Arabic Musical Scales with 2 Audio CDs:
Basic Maqam Teachings

Harmonic Secrets of Arabic Music Scales with 2 Audio CDs:
Fine Tuning the Maqams

Singing in Baghdad:
A Musical Mission of Peace

The books listed above can be ordered from:
http://www.gldesignpub.com
or write for more info:
E-Mail: distrib@gldesignpub.com